Essential Dogs

The Complete Guide To Safely Using Essential Oils On Your Dog

By Amy Joyson

© Copyright 2015 by Amy Joyson- All rights reserved.

This document is geared towards providing exact and reliable information in regards to the topic and issue covered. The publication is sold with the idea that the publisher is not required to render accounting, officially permitted, or otherwise, qualified services. If advice is necessary, legal or professional, a practiced individual in the profession should be ordered.

- From a Declaration of Principles which was accepted and approved equally by a Committee of the American Bar Association and a Committee of Publishers and Associations.

In no way is it legal to reproduce, duplicate, or transmit any part of this document in either electronic means or in printed format. Recording of this publication is strictly prohibited and any storage of this document is not allowed unless with written permission from the publisher. All rights reserved.

The information provided herein is stated to be truthful and consistent, in that any liability, in terms of inattention or otherwise, by any usage or abuse of any policies, processes, or directions contained within is the solitary and utter responsibility of the recipient reader. Under no circumstances will any legal responsibility or blame be held against the publisher for any reparation, damages, or monetary loss due to the information herein, either directly or indirectly.

Respective authors own all copyrights not held by the publisher.

The information herein is offered for informational purposes solely, and is universal as so. The presentation of the information is without contract or any type of guarantee assurance.

The trademarks that are used are without any consent, and the publication of the trademark is without permission or backing by the trademark owner. All trademarks and brands within this book are for clarifying purposes only and are the owned by the owners themselves, not affiliated with this document.

Disclaimer – Please read!

The information provided in this book is designed to provide helpful information on the subjects discussed. This book is not meant to be used, nor should it be used, to diagnose or treat any medical condition. For diagnosis or treatment of any medical problem, consult your own physician. The publisher and author are not responsible for any specific health or allergy needs that may require medical supervision and are not liable for any damages or negative consequences from any treatment, action, application or preparation, to any person reading or following the information in this book. References are provided for informational purposes only and do not constitute endorsement of any websites or other sources. Readers should be aware that the websites listed in this book may change.

Table of Contents

An Introduction to Essential Oils for Dogs..................7
Does aromatherapy for dogs exist?..8
What is the difference between hydrosols and essential oils?
....8
Is aromatherapy a safe alternative for dogs?.........................9
Different methods of using essential oils on your pet 10
Topical application of essential oils 10
Diffusion and inhalation of essential oils 11
Oral application of essential oils...11
Summary of precautions when engaging in dog aromatherapy...12

Beginners Guide to Essential Oils for Dogs..............13
Purchasing essential oils for your dog...................................13
Which essential oils are safe to begin with?........................15

Dangers to Look Out For When Using Essential Oils on Your Dog..19
So what are some of the dangers to look out for when using essential oils on your dog?..20

Does Dog Aromatherapy Work?......................................24
What does dog aromatherapy comprise of? 24
Uses of dog aromatherapy..25
How to administer essential oils effectively 26

Using Essential Oils Appropriately On Your Dog......28
Storing your essential oils 28
Prepping your dog for aromatherapy 29
Testing the essential oils..31
Reactions to look out for 32

Essential Recipes for Dog Aromatherapy...................33
Relief of arthritis related symptoms 33
Flea repellent recipe 35
Relieving anxiety 36
Eliminate bad odor from your pet..37

Tick repellent recipe..38
Eliminate hyperactivity..38
Relief from skin problems..39
Relief from ear infections...40
Treating minor wounds 41
Mosquito repellent 42
Relief from motion sickness.......................................43
Relief from sinus infections 44

2 FREE eBooks for you!

About The Author

Valerian Press

Preview Of My Book "Essential Oil Massage Techniques For Beginners"

An Introduction to Essential Oils for Dogs

Most people have heard of essential oils. However, not many know what they really are. These chemical components are naturally occurring compounds in plants. To become essential oils, they are extracted from the various plants through the process of distillation. Over the years, consistent laboratory testing have found that these compounds offer a range of benefits to both humans and pets alike. So are they are better alternative to pharmaceutical options?

Engaging in aromatherapy for pets has shown that it brings a myriad of advantages. These essential oils can be effective in treating numerous ailments that afflict dogs such as pest infestations, ear infections, skin irritations, hyperactivity and much more. In this chapter we shall look at how best to use these essential oils on your pet, as well as those that may be safe for human use but you should steer clear your dog away from.

Over the years, dog aromatherapy has started gaining momentum in pet owner circles. Nevertheless, there are still many misconceptions that people have regarding this type of new-age treatment. The first thing to note though is that aromatherapy is not a "new-age" fad. Civilizations have engaged in this practice for centuries. In addition, aromatherapy does not simply constitute lighting a bunch of candles and trying to make your dog smell nice using synthetic oils. The use of 100% hydrosols and essential oils is vital, as these are what contain the medicinal properties that will help treat the different conditions that your canine may be suffering from. By knowing what this treatment comprises of, you will be better placed at making a decision on whether a foray into aromatherapy would be the right course of action for your pet.

Does aromatherapy for dogs exist?

The answer to this is a resounding yes. Aromatherapy for dogs simple refers to the use of pure essential oils and untainted hydrosols with the aim of holistic treatment for your canine. When used appropriately, aromatherapy can treat both behavioural as well as physical conditions afflicting your pet. What you need to know off the bat is that aromatherapy is not limiting yourself to grooming products for your pet. Rather it encompasses using therapeutic grade oils, whether singularly or as a blend, to treat specific health problems or to enhance the overall wellbeing of your pet. By now, you may have noticed my consistent use of the words "therapeutic" and "100% pure". This is not for naught as for your pet to reap the health benefits of aromatherapy; you need to be certain that you are only making use of pure hydrosols and essential oils.

Opting for cheaper options that may smell the same does not cut it as these contain synthetic compounds that could end up being detrimental to the health of your pet. Additionally, the synthetic alternatives do not offer the therapeutic benefits of pure essential oils, which may cause more harm than good.

What is the difference between hydrosols and essential oils?

Let us begin with defining an essential oil. These oils are volatile substances that are formed in the sac, veins or glandular hairs of a plant. These parts are typically located in the roots, seeds, flowers, bark and even the fruit of the plant. They are considered to be the main essence of the plant and thus the compounds aptly named essential oils, as they are responsible for the unique scent of the particular plant. The essential oils are extracted in various ways.

The most common method of extraction is steam distillation. However you can also find that essential oils have been derived through carbon dioxide extraction, solvent extraction and lastly through manual expression. Contrary to their name, essential oils are actually not oily. These compounds tend to be highly concentrated thus need to be diluted before use. They are diluted in carrier oils and perhaps that is why most people make the mistake of assuming they are oily compounds. Every essential oil has its own set of distinct properties when it comes to their scent, their chemical composition, their color and more. That is why you find that different essential oils will have their own different set of healing properties. Some of the properties that a majority of them have in common though is being antibacterial, antifungal and antiviral.

A hydrosol, on the other hand, is a water-based compound that is a by-product of steam distillation of the essential oils. Hydrosols comprise of water-soluble components of the plant as well as some essential oils from the plant. Hydrosols are nowhere near as concentrated as essential oils. As such, they can be safely used without dilution. You can also opt to dilute your preferred essential oil in a hydrosol if you are looking to reap the synergistic effects of the two.

If your pet is extremely sensitive, you can opt to use hydrosols for their aromatherapy rather than essential oils, as they are a competent alternative.

Is aromatherapy a safe alternative for dogs?

By now, you know that essential oils are compounds that are highly concentrated. As such, it is safe to say they tend to be extremely potent. With that in mind, using them on your dog should be done with utmost care. Most people make the mistake of adding a few more drops of essential oil than recommended and this is when you start putting your pet at risk. Always use the recommended amount depending on the size of your dog. Moreover, essential oils should only be used in tandem with carrier oils. When diluted in the appropriate manner, essential oils will not be quite beneficial for your pet, but will also prove to be a great therapeutic option for them.

However, not all essential oils are recommended for use on your pet. Here is a quick list of different essential oils that should never be used on your dog, whether in diluted form or not.

1. Juniper wood oil: This essential oil can prove toxic to dog kidneys. However, juniper berry oil is perfectly safe for dogs.
2. Birch and wintergreen essential oils: When use on the skin of dogs, these oils can prove to be toxic. This is due to the methyl salicylate they contain. Ingesting them can cause poisoning and even death.
3. Cassia essential oil: If use on the skin this essential oil can cause dermal irritation on your dog.
4. Horseradish essential oil: Known to be quite pungent, this essential oil may be too strong for your pet's keen senses and can also cause skin irritation.
5. Wormwood essential oil: It should be noted that wormwood in both its herbal form as well as an essential oil is toxic to most pets. Studies have shown that ingestion of this plant causes renal failure in people and has been known to be a cause of seizures in dogs.
6. Melaleuca essential oil.

Different methods of using essential oils on your pet

Although essential oils come in liquid form, this does not mean that there is only one way of administering aromatherapy to your dog. Generally, there are three main ways of using essential oils on your pet.

Topical application of essential oils

This is one of the most common methods of administering essential oils. It is one of the most effective techniques as you are applying the essential oil directly onto the problematic area. The essential oil is then absorbed by the skin, enabling it to penetrate the capillaries. This carries the essential oil into the bloodstream and it can begin exerting it healing properties in minimal time. For topical application, there are different techniques that can be used. These include a massage, using a spritzer, or incorporating the essential oil into the shampoo or ointments that you use on your pet. However, just because you are applying the essential oil topically or incorporating it into a shampoo does not mean you should do it while it is still concentrated. Ensure you have diluted the essential oil in a carrier oil such as jojoba oil, olive oil or sweet almond oil are all good alternatives.

Diffusion and inhalation of essential oils

As the name suggests, inhalation is letting your dog sniff the essential oil. For this to be more effective, you can use a diffuser. A diffuser works to evaporate the essential oils. It should be left working for a period between half an hour to an hour. Your dog will be inhaling the essential oils during this period and they will get absorbed into its bloodstream. For optimal results, use a diffuser twice a day for about a week.

Oral application of essential oils

This technique of administering essential oils to your pet should be done with extreme precaution. In fact is wholly advised to ensure that this is done under the supervision of a holistic professional, as some essential oils can prove toxic to pets by simply giving them a slightly different dosage than recommended. Since these essential oils are highly concentrated, chances of an overdose are quite high especially if you are an amateur to aromatherapy for pets. It is therefore advisable for newbie enthusiast to limit themselves to the first two application techniques and leave oral application to a holistic veterinarian.

Summary of precautions when engaging in dog aromatherapy

1. Only use 100% pure essential oils that are of therapeutic grade.
2. Limit yourself to essential oils that are proven safe for dogs.
3. Always dilute essential oils in carrier oils before use.
4. Small dogs will need a lower dosage of essential oils as compared to larger dogs. It is not a one size fits all scenario.
5. If a dog is pregnant or elderly, opt for hydrosols rather than pure essential oils.
6. Do not engage in aromatherapy on dogs prone to seizures or that suffer from epilepsy.
7. Never apply essential oils close to the dog's eyes, nose or genitals.

Beginners Guide to Essential Oils for Dogs

After our first chapter, you now know that essential oils are a great alternative to treat a myriad of dog ailments. These include motion sickness, pest infestations, arthritis in older dogs and many more. However, as aforementioned, not all essential oils will be safe for use on your beloved pet. In this chapter, we shall look at the essential oils that all newbies can venture into aromatherapy with. None of these carries any side effects for your dog, while still being chock full of health benefits.

For most newbie essential oil enthusiasts, the experience can prove to be quite overwhelming. This is simply because there is a wide range of essential oils out there. So how do you know which ones to choose? How can you tell which ones to avoid? Well this is the chapter for you. Not only will we delve into what to look for when buying essential oils, but we will also reveal the first essential oils that are safe and easy to use on your pet.

Keep in mind that there are thousands of essentials oils out there. This, however, does not mean you have to invest in all of them in the name of holistic treatment for your pet. To make it easier for you, you need a must-have list of essential oils. This makes it much simpler to engage in aromatherapy for your dog, as you will not be inundating yourself with varying options. Once you become better at this type of alternative treatment, you can then start considering other options for your pet depending on how confident you are with your choices.

Purchasing essential oils for your dog

The one thing that you should never compromise when it comes to using essential oils on your pet is their authenticity. Just as we have a variety of supermarkets and products to choose from when buying every day stuff, you will also find that there are innumerable places to purchase these essential oils. In addition to this, they will also come with different price tags ranging from extremely expensive to dirt-cheap. In this instance, cheap will definitely prove to be expensive. The rule of thumb is to only use therapeutic grade oils on your pets. This are one hundred percent pure and thus do not expect them to come cheap. So what should you look out for if you are buying essential oils for the first time?

1. Buy essential oils that are packaged in glass bottles. Moreover, the bottles should be violet, cobalt or amber in color. This is to prevent the essential oils from reacting to light exposure. However, always ensure that when storing the bottles you keep them in a dark and dry place.

2. Read the information on the packaging. You should know a few things before purchasing the essential oil of your choice. Look out for: the scientific name, the generic name, the method of extraction, how the plant was cultivated and the country of origin.

3. Ensure that the packaging clearly states that the essential oil is "100% pure".

4. Resist the urge to save some money by buying the cheaper options. Remember, you do not have to buy an entire collection of essential oils right off the bat. Instead, you can slowly cultivate your collection as time goes on. With this is mind, never purchase the cheaper alternative as more often than not, they tend to be adulterated versions of pure essential oils. Some of them are even purely synthetic and could end up doing more harm than good on your pet.

5. Always buy essential oils from a holistic vendor. You may come across these oils at your local supermarket or

food store. However, these tend to be of a different quality than those sold holistic centres. To be on the safe side, always purchase your first batch from a well-known holistic treatment centre.

Which essential oils are safe to begin with?

Bergamot essential oil
This essential oil is known for its antifungal and soothing properties. It is best used to treat ear infections that have sprung up due to either bacteria or a yeast infection. Take note though that bergamot causes photosensitivity to dogs. As such, ensure that your pet avoids the sun right after application. To be on the safe side you could choose to only apply bergamot on your pet at night.

Carrot seed essential oil
This essential oil has anti-inflammatory properties. It can also be used as a mild antibacterial. It works great on pets who have sensitive, flaky skin that is prone to infections. It works by stimulating the regeneration of tissues on the dermis. It is also great for the healing of scars on your pet.

Cedar wood essential oil
The properties exhibited by this essential oil include stimulating circulation and being an anti-inflammatory. This makes it a good option for ridding your dog of a flea infestation. Cedar wood can be safely applied on both the dog's coat as well as their dermis.

German Chamomile essential oil
This essential oil has both non-toxic as well as anti-inflammatory properties. German chamomile is great for treating skin irritations that your dog may be experiencing. It is also a good choice for treating any allergic reactions that may exhibit themselves on the skin. You can use German chamomile to soothe burns too.

Roman Chamomile essential oil

The properties contained in this essential oil include being an antispasmodic and an analgesic. This means it is best suited for treating conditions pertaining to the central nervous system. Being an analgesic, it is a good option for pain relief in muscle, toothache in your pet a well as cramps.

Sage

This essential oil mainly works to calm the nerves of your pet. When diluted appropriately it can be used as a sedative on your dog's central nervous system.

Eucalyptus

This essential oil has both anti-inflammatory and anti-viral properties. However, it is best known as an expectorant in both humans as well as animals. For that reason, it is a good option for relieving chest congestion in your pet. However, it can also be effective as a flea repellent due to its pungent scent.

Geranium essential oil

The main property in this is essential oil is it being anti-fungal, Thus it serves as a good treatment opting for ear infections and skin irritations that have been caused by fungi. Geranium essential oil can also be used as a tick repellent on your dog's coat.

Ginger essential oil

In humans, ginger is known as a good digestion aid. The same is true in dogs and it can also help abate motion sickness in your pet. The mild analgesic properties in ginger can also work toward effective pain relief in your dog if the pet suffers from arthritis or dysplasia.

Helichrysum essential oil

This essential oil is considered extremely therapeutic with its regenerative properties as well as being anti-inflammatory and a mild analgesic. It can be applied topically to relieve skin irritations your dog may be suffering from such as eczema. It is also effective in the soothing of bruises and eventual healing of scars. Helichrysum can also be used for mild pain relief in your per due to its analgesic properties.

Lavender essential oil

This essential oil is known for its calming effects and that is why it is used in a range of human products. However, it also has anti-bacterial properties and can prevent itching in pets. This makes it a great option when treating skin irritations making it one of the best starter oils when venturing into pet aromatherapy.

Sweet marjoram essential oil

This essential oil is not only a soothing muscle relaxant, but it also contains strong antibacterial properties. As such, sweet marjoram is the go-to essential oil when trying to rid your pet of bacterial skin infections. It is also a good insect repellent if your dog is suffering from a pest infestation.

Niaouli essential oil

The properties of this essential oil include being both anti-itch and anti-bacterial. It can also be used to calm your dog's nerves though a gentle massage. Niaouli essential oil would be a great choice if you were looking to treat bacterial infections on the dermis. It also can be used to combat a range of skin infections that come about due to pet allergies.

Peppermint essential oil

The properties that this essential oil contains include being antispasmodic and insect repelling due to its scent. It is also known to be great for stimulating circulation making it a good treatment option to relieve the symptoms of arthritis in dogs.

When travelling with your pet, you can use it in tandem with ginger as a method of treating motion sickness.

Valerian essential oil

This essential oil is known for its calming properties. When diluted appropriately you can administer it to your pet to treat different forms of anxiety.

By no means is this a conclusive list of all the essential oils that would be great for your pet. However, they are a good place to start for individuals who are looking to test the waters when it comes to aromatherapy for their pet.

Dangers to Look Out For When Using Essential Oils on Your Dog

With aromatherapy breaking conventional barriers, more pet owners are opting for this type of therapy for at home use. However, this does not result in exclusively positive results. For pet owners who have not conducted the appropriate research, pets have become harmed and even succumbed to death due to negligence. For instance, the essential oil Melaleuca has received a lot of notoriety in recent times. For one, it I widely available for human use. In humans, it can be used to treat skin disorders stemming from bites or scratches. Pet owners who have opted to use this on their furry friends have realize that just because it is suitable for human use does not automatically mean it is the best option for animals. Pets who have had this essential oil applied on them for dermatological reasons will end up exhibiting symptoms related to toxicity. These symptoms include depression, ataxia, lack of coordination, vomiting and involuntary tremors.

The biggest cause for these unfortunate circumstances is misinformation. We can concur that these pet owners are simply trying to provide the best holistic care for their animals. However, if you are unaware of the dangers posed by certain essential oils, then you end up harming your pet. That is why it is important to discern the essential oils that are safe for humans while being unsafe for pets and vice versa. Another good example of this is Pennyroyal essential oil. If ingested by humans, this essential oil can cause liver and kidney failure as it acts as an abortifacient. On the other hand, this essential oil is a good flea repellent on pets!

It should also be noted that just because certain essential oils are good for your dog, does not mean that they should also be administered to your other pets. Let us take a look at cats for instance. A large number of products that are used on cats contain marginal amounts of essential oils. If you are using a range of products on your cat, you will find that over time toxins may end up building up in your feline's system. If this goes unchecked, it could lead to eventual organ failure. This is because a cat does not process toxins at nearly the same rate as a dog does. In addition, dogs still process these toxins much less effectively than humans do. Chemical compounds such as phenols, ketones and more can be found in some of the essential oils. The effects from regular exposure to them can take weeks, months or even years to materialize.

This is not the end of your pet aromatherapy journey through.

Granted, knowing that the chance of error is high can seem quite daunting to individuals who are simply testing the waters of dog aromatherapy. Nevertheless, the cautions are not in place to put the fear of all things aromatherapeutic in you. Instead knowing how vulnerable your pet can be should instil a sense of responsibility when it comes to selecting the appropriate essential oil for them. Being knowledgeable before embarking on this endeavour will eliminate a great deal of the risk surrounding using any and all essential oils on your pet.

So what are some of the dangers to look out for when using essential oils on your dog?

Not picking the right oils
One of the biggest concerns you should have when making a selection of essential oils for your dog is the purity. This can never be stressed enough. For instance, it takes about a hundred pounds of lavender to produce a single pound of its essential. With this in mind, it should not be surprising that essential oils should cost a bit on the higher side. However, some brands make themselves more marketable by diluting the essential oil in other substances, which will leave it smelling the same, but could end up having adverse effects on your pet. Worse still there is a range of synthetic essential oils that are sold in the market and these are purely for fragrance purposes, as they do not have the innate healing properties of one hundred percent pure essential oil. If you are choosing

essential oils specifically for pet aromatherapy, always double check that what you are buying is a hundred percent pure. How can you go about this?
1. Feel the texture. As aforementioned, despite their name, essential oils are not greasy to the touch.
2. Read the fine print on the packaging.
3. Be wary of throwaway prices.

Using the wrong oils

Ensuring that you get a hundred percent pure essential oils is just one of the things to look out for. The next would be to watch out that you are not using the wrong essential oils on your pet. The essential oils may be legitimate but if they are not suited for dogs, then your pet will suffer an adverse reaction. Always keep in mind that a product being all-natural does not always translate into it being safe. Some of the essential oils that should never be in close proximity to your pet include:
1. Clove
2. Horseradish
3. Anise
4. Juniper
5. Wintergreen
6. Thyme
7. Yarrow
8. Melaleuca
9. Pennyroyal

These are just the tip of the iceberg, as we cannot create a fully comprehensive list. As such, it goes without saying that before you contemplate using an essential oil on your dog, conduct sufficient research beforehand to ensure that it will be safe for your pet.

Administering the essential oils inappropriately

So you have confirmed that your essential oils are a hundred percent pure and that they are safe for use on your dog. This does not mean you are fully in the clear though. Some pet owners put their furry friends at risk by simply administering the essential oils in the wrong manner. Here are some of the things to keep in mind when you are attempting to engage in pet aromatherapy on your own.

1. Always dilute the essential oil in a carrier oil. The general rule of thumb for pets is 25% of the ratio you would use for humans. However, it is always good to get specific instructions from your holistic veterinarian.
2. Never administer essential oils to your pet orally. Although some of the essential oils will only be effective through this mode, it is not advisable for pet owners to do this on their own. If the situation calls for it, enlist the services of your holistic veterinarian.
3. Do not use essential oils on pregnant dogs, puppies under the age of ten weeks and elderly dogs. For these groups of pets, opt for the use of hydrosols, as they are less potent than their essential oil counterparts are.
4. Keep a keen eye on your pet. Remember, your dog cannot tell you if they are having an adverse reaction to the essential oil, you need to look out for any abnormal behaviour such as whining, constant sniffing, regular scratching and any other sign that may be out of the ordinary.
5. Introduce the essential oils gradually. Do not jump both feet first when venturing into pet aromatherapy. Give your dog some time to get used to the scent by starting off with small doses of applications once a day.
6. Watch out for sensitive body parts. Never let the essential oils come close to your dog's eyes, mouth, genitalia and nose. Especially the nose since this is one of the most sensitive senses on your canine.

As an animal lover, your best bet would be to thoroughly educate yourself before engaging in any form of aromatherapy on your dog. While doing so, you should also keep in mind that misinformation is widespread too. It is always best advised to run what you know by your holistic veterinarian first to ensure that you are on the right track.

Does Dog Aromatherapy Work?

After reading about the hazards of improper use of essential oils as well as the safety precautions that all pet owners should adhere to, you may now be wondering if this treatment option is worth all the fuss. One thing we can agree on is that aromatherapy has been found to be effective in humans. Due to the antiseptic and antimicrobial effects of these oils, they have been use for centuries by humans to detoxify their system and regulate their circulation. Ancient civilizations such as the Chinese, the Greeks and even the ancient Egyptian has an extensive understanding on how these aromatic plants work. Thus used them for centuries toward their own health benefits. Although their application in the canine realm is fairly new, it is safe to say that interest in dog aromatherapy is growing in leaps and bounds. A large number of modern vets are hopping onto the bandwagon as they become more knowledgeable of the benefits of herbal remedies, aromatherapy and acupuncture to our furry friends. There are even some pet insurance companies that include these treatments in their packages. The question remains, does this treatment really work?

What does dog aromatherapy comprise of?

When it comes to dog aromatherapy, the main course of treatment here is stimulating your pet's limbic system. This is the section of your dog's brain that is responsible for controlling the pet's moods as well as their emotions. This is why you will find that dog aromatherapy is one of the most effective ways of ridding your pet of feelings associate with anxiety, fear, stress, anger and more.

The therapeutic oils can be administered in various ways for maximum efficacy. The three main ways this is done is through topical application on the skin, inhalation and professionally they can be administered orally. These oils can either be administered one at a time or a blend can be used depending on what you are trying to achieve. Generally, they should evoke feelings of sedation, pain relief, calming, re-energizing, rejuvenation and more.

Uses of dog aromatherapy

As aforementioned, one of the main uses it to provide a calming effect for your dog without the use of drugs. Take for instance during Fourth of July. At this time, many pets get agitated due to the constant fireworks an excessive noise that is usually not part of their daily routine. The loud bangs can invoke feelings of anxiety in your pet and some dogs may even become aggressive. Making use of dog aromatherapy can enable them to be calm and relaxed. They are also a great option for combatting hyperactivity in your pet, aggression, separation anxiety and other psychological ailments.

Nevertheless, this is not their only use. Topical application of essential oils can also treat a range of skin ailments such as rashes or skin irritations. These also will include the treatment of skin ailments that stem from allergic reactions.

Essential oils can be sued as a repellent. A host of them have been known to be effective in ridding dogs of fleas and ticks. However, they can also be used to repel other insects such as mosquitoes and flies.

Essential oils are a great alternative for older dogs who may be suffering from joint aches or arthritis. By stimulating your dog's circulation, they can expect to feel some relief after application. They can also be used in younger dogs to relieve growing pains. However, you should note that the use of essential oils on both puppies and older dogs should be done only when they have been sufficiently diluted. Alternatively you could opt to use hydrosols instead as these categories of dogs wold be more sensitive to the essential oils.

Aside from immediate relief, essential oils can also be used on your dog as a preventative measure. This would be a way of ensuring that the different systems in their body remain healthy, thus avoiding any major medical emergencies. This includes preventative care for their immune system, their digestive system, their liver and more.

How to administer essential oils effectively

When it comes to administering essential oils to your pet, you always have to remember that their sense of smell is hundreds of times stronger than ours. A dog's nose has been known to contain millions of scent receptors. Millions! As such, once they inhale the essential oils it is passed on to their bloodstream in record time. For this reason, you will find that aromatherapy on your pet will be quite fast acting making it an efficient alternative when contemplating how to treat a certain health condition.

When applying the essential oils topically, do not simply pour the oils on your dog and let them be. For effective use, ensure you give your dog a proper massage when engaging in topical application. For better results, you could opt to target specific areas on your pet's body. Some of the places that are suitable for topical application for effective results include the joints of their limbs, their spine and lastly a good old belly rub. When rubbing these essential oils on your dog's belly, take measures to avoid their genitalia as this could prove quite uncomfortable for your pet. Additionally, to make the most of topical application of these essential oils, try your best to concentrate on the parts of their body that have minimal hair. For one, this will prevent your dog having to deal with an oily coat. Secondly, the less hair that is in the way, the easier it will be for the essential oils to penetrate the skin. You can also consider incorporating the essential oils into your pet's hygiene routine. This means mixing the recommended dose into their shampoo or conditioner.

Lastly, when it comes to inhalation, it is not advisable to simply put the bottle of essential oil under their nose and have them sniff it. As mentioned earlier, dogs have millions of scent receptors and this could prove to be overwhelming for them. Instead, invest in a diffuser that you can use for this specific task. These diffusers work almost the same as the plug-in air conditioners. Once you have appropriately mixed the essential oils, pour the liquid into a diffuser and plug it into a power socket. Have the dog in the room for several hours as the diffuser releases tiny particles over that period of time. This will make it easier for the pet to breathe in the essential oil.

In conclusion

Lastly, remember that dog aromatherapy is not something that should be taken lightly. If you are a newbie, you need to ensure that you have as much research as possible so as to avoid harming your pet. It is always advisable to seek the counsel of a holistic veterinarian before engaging in any treatments on your dog. Not only will this allow you to know your limits for pet aromatherapy, but you also get first hand advice on how best to mix the essential oils whether it is in carrier oils or if you are making a blend. At the end of the day, this course of treatment is supposed to heal your dog and not make them more ill. In the event that you notice the course of treatment is not being effective, you should always seek medical advice from a vet rather than starting a new course of aromatherapy treatment on your pet.

Using Essential Oils Appropriately On Your Dog

By now, we know just as with other commercial products, you can also find the essential oil market flooded with fakes and unoriginal products. These synthetic imitations may seem like a way of cost cutting, but they pose numerous dangers to your pet. For one, they may not even work in the first place meaning they will simply be a waste of money. However, these synthetic and fake alternatives have also been known to cause a host of negative side effects on pets. Some even leading to death. One mistake you should never do as a pet owner is mistakenly choose fragrance oils as an alternative to essential oils. Fragrance oils are synthetic aromatic versions of essential oils whose main purpose is to make a room smell nice. They have no therapeutic properties whatsoever. So what should you look for when purchasing essential oils?

Things to look out for on the packaging
1. The batch number of the essential oil.
2. The botanical name of the essential oil.
3. The layman name of the essential oil.
4. Its organic certification.
5. Date of bottling of the essential oil.

Things to enquire about at the store
1. The method of extraction used to get the essential oil.
2. The plant parts used in the extraction.
3. The country of origin of the essential oil.

Storing your essential oils

Another way that you can spot counterfeit oils and the real deal is through how they are stored. Pure essential oils come in bottles that are tinted in a dark color. These dark colored bottles could be either amber, green or blue. In addition to this, the essential oils should only be stored in a cool and dark place. This is to increase their shelf life by avoiding exposure to sunlight. One thing to note though that the healing properties of essential oils will diminish over time. This does not mean that they will become worthless though. Essential oils that have been shelved for years at a time may not still be therapeutically effective but they will sustain their strong fragrance. You can then use them for their aroma around the home rather than for their healing properties. Never store your essential oils in a plastic container or one made from steel. If you spot oils being sold in these types of packaging, chances are they are synthetic. Over time, the essential oils will melt the plastic container and could end up reacting with the minerals in the steel.

Prepping your dog for aromatherapy

When it comes to the administration of essential oils, you should not just jump right in to the process. Instead, form a connection with your pet so that they can feel safe and secure. Having them relaxed during the process will ensure that the administration will go on without a hitch. So how can you prep your pet for this type of treatment?

1. Locate a spot where your dog feels at ease. This could be their favourite area to relax in or the spot that they usually sleep at night. The place should be familiar to them.
2. Take a moment of quiet sitting with your dog. At this time you can pet them down to make them feel more at ease. Do not use this type to play though as this could make them excitable.
3. Rub the essential oil into your hands. Ensure that you have diluted it appropriately for the size and age of your dog. Rubbing the essential oil into your hands will give your dog a moment to get familiar with the scent.
4. Start massaging the essential oil on your dog. It is best to do this in the areas that have less fur such as the belly or inner thigh. However if your dog is suffering from a

specific ache such as arthritis in their joints, then focus your attention on these parts.

Making a ritual of taking some time out with your dog before application will make it easier for them to get used to this routine. This will make the entire process pleasurable for both you and your pet.

Topical application of essential oils on your dog

When it comes to the topical application of essential oils, it cannot be stressed enough the importance of ensuring they are appropriately diluted beforehand. There are three main carrier oils that work well with almost any essential oil. These include virgin coconut oil, soybean oil and extra virgin olive oil. However, it should be noted that these are not the only carrier oils that can be used effectively. This is a good time to note that there a few exceptions of essential oils that can be applied directly. These are true lavender and chamomile essential oil. However, since we are talking about topical application on dogs, you still need to take precaution due to how sensitive their senses are. A rule of thumb if you are new to this type of treatment though is to never use any undiluted essential oils on your pet. Other measures to take in regards to safety when topically applying these essential oils is to avoid sensitive areas on your dog's body. Keep application a safe distance away from their eyes and their genitalia. Moreover, when applying the essential oils on furless areas, you need to ensure that you are not being overzealous. Keep in mind that since these areas are hairless, the skin is probably more sensitive as compared to other parts of the body.

Inhalation of essential oils

As with topical application, care should also be taken when making your dog inhale essential oils. There are several ways that aromatherapy can be administered in this way. The first would be to let your pet sniff the essential straight out the bottle. However, as convenient as this may be it is also easy to end up getting some drops on their nose and this would not fare well. A safer method would be to opt to add a few drops of essential oil on a cloth. One or two drops would be sufficient for this. Your pet can then sniff the cloth intermittently. Lastly, the most effective method of administering these oils using inhalation would be through a diffuser. All that would be required of you is to ensure that your pet stays in the room for the duration that the diffuser will be switched on.

Ingestion of essential oils

For people venturing into pet aromatherapy for the first time, this is not recommended. However, if you have had some practice, you will find that some essential oils work best when they are administered orally. The essential oils can either be mixed in the dog's food or given to them directly after being mixed with honey or a carrier oil. Before engaging in this though, you need to have a go ahead from your holistic veterinarian who will undoubtedly provide you with the appropriate steps of doing so.

Remember, before any administration of the essential oils, you should take the time to introduce it to your pet. Let them have a whiff of it and gauge their reaction, as most animals will inherently know what is safe for them or not. Additionally, letting them become familiar with the fragrance will make it easier to engage in the aromatherapy.

Testing the essential oils

Before embarking on any aromatherapeutic treatment, it is pertinent to perform a test on your dog first. Although most approved essential oils will not cause an adverse reaction, you need to keep in mind that each dog is unique. Your particular pet either may be excessively sensitive or perhaps has an inherent reaction with a specific essential oil. With this in mind, perform a patch test at least 24 hours prior. All you need to do is apply a small amount of the mixed essential oil on a visible part of their body. If they have not developed a rash or any swelling on the spot once the test window is done, then chances are they will not suffer any allergic reaction to the essential oil. However, in the event that your pet does show signs of reacting to the patch test, simply thoroughly wipe off the essential oil. This will be most effectively done when you use a carrier oil such as extra virgin olive oil. After getting the essential oil off, wipe down the area a second time with some warm water.

Reactions to look out for

As mentioned in previous chapters, there is a range of essential oils that should never be used on your pet. However, the list is by no means exhaustive and as a pet owner, you should always take measures to ensure the type of essential oil you are contemplating is safe for your pet. Nevertheless, nothing is ever a hundred percent sure. There are a number of variables that could affect whether your pet ends up having an adverse reaction. The first would be human error by opting for the wrong essential oil. Other variables include the weight of the pet, any health conditions, the sensitivity of your pet, the breed of your dog and more. So what are some of the reactions to look out or that could indicate your pet is not handling the aromatherapy well?

1. Heavy breathing
2. Lethargy
3. Exhibiting distress

These reactions ten to occur if an essential oil contraindicates a pre-existing ailment your pet may be suffering from. Alternatively, perhaps the blend is simply too strong for your dog especially if they did not fail the patch test. Overall, utmost care must be taken and in the event of an adverse reaction, seek immediate veterinary care for your pet.

Essential Recipes for Dog Aromatherapy

Now that you are relatively versed on the benefits of aromatherapy on your dog, as well as have an understanding on the precautions to take to avoid the wrong use of them, we can now delve into recipes that could come in handy for your pet. As always, keep in mind your dog's initial reaction to the essential oils. Never forget to mix them with carrier oils unless stated otherwise. Moreover, always perform a patch test 24 hours prior to application.

Relief of arthritis related symptoms

There are two different blends that you could use to treat the symptoms of arthritis. Your choice would depend on the essential oils that you have available as they both work toward offering the same type of relief.

Massage oil 1
Ingredients
- 15ml of olive oil
- 2 drops ginger essential oil
- 3 drops of valerian essential oil
- 4 drops of peppermint essential oil
- 6 drops of helichrysum essential oil

Massage oil 2
Ingredients
- 15ml sweet almond oil
- 2 drops of lavender essential oil
- 3 drops of ginger essential oil
- 4 drops of rosemary essential oil

Method
Use either of the two recipes to concoct an arthritis blend. Once you have mixed the ingredients appropriately, massage

the recipes into your dog's limbs. You can also apply a drop or two of the blend onto each ear tip.

Flea repellent recipe

Ingredients
- ➤ 3 drops lemon essential oil
- ➤ 2 drops citronella essential oil
- ➤ 4 drops clary sage essential oil
- ➤ 8 drops peppermint essential oil

Method
With this recipe, you have the option of either mixing the blend with a carrier oil or simply integrating it into your dog's shampoo. If you would prefer applying it with a base oil, it is recommended to mix the ingredients into 15ml of virgin olive oil or jojoba oil. If used in a shampoo, ensure that the shampoo you are using is all-natural. Additionally, this blend will only be enough for 240 ml of shampoo at a time. When using this recipe with a carrier oil, apply the blend to the pet's legs, neck, chest, back and tail. Including a few drops of this blend (in the carrier oil) on the dog's collar can also work toward repelling fleas.

Relieving anxiety

Many dogs suffer from different forms of anxiety ranging from noise anxiety, separation anxiety from their owner, a fear of strange places and more. Two recipes can be used to relieve this.

Massage Blend 1
Ingredients
- 15ml jojoba oil
- 2 drops clary sage essential oil
- 3 drops sweet marjoram essential oil
- 3 drops valerian essential oil
- 5 drops lavender essential oil

Method
Rub 3 drops of the blend between your hands until it becomes warm then gently rub it between your pet's toes, on their outer ears and on the dog's inner thighs.

Powder blend 2
Ingredients
- 1 drop of ylang ylang essential oil
- 2 drops of Melissa essential oil
- 3 drops of lavender essential oil
- 2 drops of bergamot essential oil

Method
With this recipe, you will mix the blend into some powder to make a powdery consistency. The best options for this include corn-starch, baking soda or some rice flour. Take note that with this recipe, we are not using a carrier oil, as the powder will act as the "base oil". Put the blend into one cup of the flour you have chosen then mix well. This powder can then be sprinkled onto a safety blanket or on the dog's bed or cage to calm its nerves.

Eliminate bad odor from your pet

There are a couple of recipes that are effective in ridding your dog of bad odor. This can range from the dog's regular body odour or perhaps you would like to eliminate the wet dog smell on a rainy day.

Blend 1
Ingredients
- 3 drops of sweet marjoram essential oil
- 2 drops of geranium essential oil
- 2 drops of Roman chamomile essential oil
- 8 drops of lavender essential oil

Method

Mix this blend into 240ml of your dog's shampoo before giving them a bath. Ensure that the shampoo is all-natural.

Blend 2
Ingredients
- 1 cup of distilled water
- 3 drops of eucalyptus essential oil
- 6 drops of orange essential oil
- 6 drops of peppermint essential oil
- 10 drops of lavender essential oil

Method

In this blend, the distilled water will act as your carrier oil. Thoroughly mix all the ingredients in a spray bottle. You can then choose to spritz your of with this spray. However, you have to be careful not to get any of it on the pet's nose, eyes, genitalia and other sensitive areas. It should be strictly applied on its coat. A general rule of thumb would be to completely avoid its head and nether regions.

Tick repellent recipe

Ingredients
- 15ml of extra virgin olive oil or sweet almond oil
- 3 drops of bay leaf essential oil
- 5 drops of geranium essential oil
- 7 drops of lavender essential oil

Method
Apply a couple of drops of this blend on your dog's tail, back, neck, chest and legs.

Eliminate hyperactivity

Ingredients
- 15ml of jojoba oil or sweet almond oil
- 2 drops of roman chamomile essential oil
- 2 drops of bergamot essential oil
- 3 drops of valerian essential oil
- 3 drops of sweet marjoram essential oil
- 5 drops of lavender essential oil

Method
Rub 3 drops of this blend into your hand before topical application in between your dog's toes and on the edge of its ears.

Relief from skin problems

Ingredients
- 2 drops of German chamomile essential oil
- 3 drops of carrot seed essential oil
- 3 drops of geranium essential oil
- 7 drops of lavender essential oil

Method
There are two ways that you can make use of this blend. The first would be mixing it with 15ml of your preferred carrier oil and use it to massage into the problem areas. The second would be to mix it with 240ml of an all-natural shampoo and give your dog a bath. If your dog were suffering from itchy skin, making an oil blend using jojoba carrier oil would be a good option.

Relief from ear infections

This blend is both preventative as well as a treatment option. Apply it every time you have cleaned out your dog's ears.

Ingredients
- 15ml of virgin olive oil or sweet almond oil
- 2 drops of tea tree oil
- 3 drops of roman chamomile essential oil
- 4 drops of lavender essential oil
- 7 drops of bergamot essential oil

Method

Since this blend can be used over a long period of time, ensure you mix the ingredients in a dark colored glass bottle. You can then administer 2 drops of the blend into each ear canal and follow this up by a gentle massage on your dog's outer ear. After letting it sit for a few minutes, you will find that the oil blend will have loosened any dirt present. This makes it easier for you to clean the air with a cotton ball. The cleaner your pet's ears are, the less prone to infections they will be. Additionally, the antibacterial properties of the lavender and the antiviral properties of the tea tree oil with stimulate the healing of any infection.

Treating minor wounds

This oil blend is handy for minor scrapes, insect bites and bruises.

Ingredients
- 15ml of sweet almond oil or jojoba oil
- 1 drop of helichrysum essential oil
- 2 drops of niaouli essential oil
- 3 drops of sweet marjoram essential oil
- 4 drops of lavender essential oil

Method

Once mixed, store this blend in a dark glass bottle in your dog's first aid kit. This blend should not be massaged into the wound area though but simply apply a couple of drops on the wound site.

Mosquito repellent

This recipe comes in handy especially during the summer when mosquitoes becomes insufferable. It has also been known to ward of fleas as they are repulsed by the smell.

Ingredients
- 8oz of aloe vera juice
- 10 drops of myrrh essential oil
- 10 drops of lemongrass essential oil
- 10 drops of rose geranium essential oil
- 20 drops of citronella essential oil

Method
In this blend, the aloe vera juice acts as your carrier oil. Mix this in a spray bottle and shake thoroughly. Spritz this evenly on your dog's coat avoiding any contact with its head and nether regions.

Relief from motion sickness

This blend works toward calming your pet's stomach if it is upset due to motion sickness

Ingredients
- 15ml of virgin olive oil
- 6 drops of ginger essential oil
- 8 drops of peppermint essential oil

Method

Mix the blend then gently rub it into your dog's armpits, on their belly and at the tips of their ears. If you are taking a long drive, you can also apply this on a cotton ball and place the ball on the air vents in the car.

Relief from sinus infections

Sinus infections tend to be quite uncomfortable for dogs as they end up suffering from nasal congestion. This blend relieves this enabling them to breathe better.

Ingredients
- 15ml of sweet almond oil
- 5 drops of ravensare essential oil
- 5 drops of eucalyptus essential oil
- 5 drops of myrrh essential oil

Method
Once you have mixed the blend, topically massage a couple of drops on your dog's neck and chest. For continuous relief, you can add a couple of drops onto a bandanna and loosely tie this as a collar. This blend can also be used in tandem with a humidifier to enable your dog's chest to decongest faster. A diffuser would also work well for this purpose.

2 FREE eBooks for you!

Guys, thanks so much for reading my book. I truly hope it served as a great introduction to lavender essential oil. As a token of appreciation I have prepared two free ebooks for you. Here is a bit of information about them!

The 10 Most Important Essential Oils

In this book we delve deep into the uses and applications of the ten essential oils that I consider to be the most 'essential'. For each oil I explain the key health benefits, teach you the therapeutic applications and provide specific safety precaution. I include one of my most useful remedies for each of the oils as well. So you will receive a deep knowledge of ten essential oils and ten brilliant remedies for free! It is a 10k word eBook, the same length as this one!

When you receive this ebook you will also receive a couple of emails from me a week containing even more information about the essential oils! I will endeavor to give you at least 5 recipes or remedies per week and also provide you with some great information on the lesser known essential oils.

Simply click here to receive the ebooks!
Or type this link into a web browser: http://bit.ly/1EuHgyn

The Ultimate Guide To Vitamins

This is another wonderful 10k word ebook that has been made available to you through my publisher, Valerian Press. As a health conscious person you should be well aware of the uses and health benefits of each of the vitamins that should make up our diet. This book gives you an easy to understand, scientific explanation of the vitamin followed by the recommended daily dosage. It then highlights all the important health benefits of each vitamin. A list of the best sources of each vitamin is provided and you are also given some actionable next steps for each vitamin to make sure you are utilizing the information!

As well as receiving the free ebooks you will also be sent a weekly stream of free ebooks, again from my publishing company Valerian Press. You can expect to receive at least a new, free ebook each and every week. Sometimes you might receive a massive 10 free books in a week!

Simply click here to receive the ebooks!
Or type this link into a web browser: http://bit.ly/1EuHgyn

About The Author

Hey there! I'm Amy Joyson, a lifelong student of holistic and alternative medicine. My journey began as far back as I can remember, my mother, a practicing aromatherapist, taught me value of natural remedies as a youngster. I don't think I could imagine a life without the essential oils if I tried, they are just so important to me. I am passionate about sharing their value with as many people as possible, which led me to writing my books. If you have read any of my books I truly hope they have added value to your life and I thank you with all my heart for trusting in me.

Outside of being an author, I work as a personal trainer. Employing my deep knowledge of alternative treatments has enabled me to provide outstanding results for all of my clients!

In my spare time you will often find me lounging in my hammock reading the latest aromatherapy magazine or romantic fiction novel. I have a soft spot for true romance! I aim to meditate at least once a day, and practice yoga 5 times a week. My biggest hobby however is exploring the beautiful world that we live in. Next on my hit list is Iceland, there is something seriously alluring about that island.

You can find me here on Facebook: https://www.facebook.com/pages/Amy-Joyson/435155886642915

You can find me here on Twitter: https://twitter.com/Amy_Joyson

Valerian Press

At Valerian Press we have three key beliefs.

Providing outstanding value: We believe in enriching all of our customers' lives, doing everything we can to ensure the best experience.

Championing new talent: We believe in showcasing the worlds emerging talent by giving them the platform to grow.

Simplicity and efficiency: We understand how valuable your time is. Our products are stream-lined and consist only of what you want. You will find no fluff with us.

We hope you have enjoyed reading Amy's guide to curing allergies.

We would love to offer you a regular supply of our free and discounted books. We cover a huge range of non-fiction genres; diet and cookbooks, health and fitness, alternative and holistic medicine, spirituality and plenty more.

All you need to do is simply click here!
Alternatively you can type this link into your web browser: http://bit.ly/18hmup4

Preview Of My Book "Essential Oil Massage Techniques For Beginners"

Chapter 4 –Stress relief

Stress is one of the most debilitating and prolific health risks in society today. There is a proven and commonly accepted link between stress and poor health, yet many of us accept stress as just a part of our everyday lives. Our fast paced, high stakes, 'always on' world means that there is little (if any!) down time in many people's day-to-day schedules. Sadly, it is not an uncommon experience to feel as though you are holding on by your fingernails as life whips around you, while telling yourself that the one or two weeks of holiday planned in the distant future will be enough to keep you sane for another year. Fortunately, even though we may not be able to do a lot to change the things causing stress in our lives, we can take some steps to minimize the natural stress response of our bodies. There is perhaps no better way to calm one's nerves and elevated stress levels, than with a long, relaxing massage. As mentioned above, human touch can be highly effective in making us feel calm, a fact which is made possible through the hormonal chemistry of the human body. Prolonged touch between two people has been shown stimulate the release of the bonding chemical, oxytocin. This hormone is released in high doses through events in which human contact typically occurs, including hugging, kissing, sex and even light touch between two people. Most interestingly, at least when it comes to controlling our stress levels, oxytocin has been shown to have a *suppressant* effect on the body's stress hormone, cortisol. So that means that the more we expose ourselves to physical interactions with other people, the less cortisol induced stress we are likely to feel. When the stress relieving properties of certain essential oils are added into the mix, massage can provide a much needed reprieve for even the most cortisol stricken individuals. We'll now take a look at some of the most effective oils, blends and treatments for stress relief through the combination of aromatherapy and massage.

One of the best essential oils for inducing feelings of calm is lavender. Lavender is great for a whole range of therapeutic conditions – in fact, it is an absolutely *essential* essential oil. There are lots of essential oils that have loads of excellent and varied remedial properties, however, lavender is really queen when it comes to the world of aromatherapy. It is wonderfully versatile and can be applied for a range of purposes: from disinfecting wounds, to burns treatment, to pain relief. It is also one of the very few essential oils that can safely be applied to the skin 'neat' or undiluted. In summary, if you had to choose a 'desert island' essential oil, lavender should naturally be the go to option! Not least among the valued properties of lavender, is its ability to be utilized as an effective treatment for stress relief. Thanks to the versatility of lavender, we'll talk more about this special oil later on, but for now it is important to remember – *lavender is great for inducing a sense of calm.* Clary sage is another essential oil that has a particularly good effect in calming a patient's nerves. Derived from the steam distilled buds and leaves of the Clary Sage plant (*Salvea Sclarea*), this essential oil exhibits many parallel and complementary properties to lavender, especially when it comes to inducing a calmative effect. This remarkable herb has long been valued in its own right for its many and varied medicinal qualities, including its effect as an antidepressant, sedative and nervine agent. Care should be taken when using clary sage in combination with alcohol, as the herb can intensify the effects of this drug. Finally, geranium oil has been shown to be a highly effective emotional 'balancing' agent, which can greatly assist those suffering from anxiety or depression.

With the above calm inducing essential oils in mind, we'll now take a look at how to combine these into a great massage blend for stress relief. When making a blend for stress relief, it is perfectly acceptable to use a fairly neutral carrier oil, such as grapeseed as the primary constituent. This is because the essential oils are really doing the lion's share of the work here, and work in two distinct ways to create a feeling of calm. First, the scent of the essential oils works through the body's olfactory system to stimulate the limbic system, and helps to regulate impulses from the central nervous system that lead to an overactive adrenal response. For this reason, a carrier oil with a relatively neutral scent should be used here. The volatile compounds of the active essential oils also work by entering the body through the bloodstream; from here, they circulate throughout the body where they can relax muscles and also influence cortisol and adrenaline levels in the body by limiting overactive stress hormone production. As such, opting for a carrier oil with a moderately good rate of absorption (such as grapeseed or apricot kernel oils) is recommended.

With this in mind, the following treatment makes for a good remedy when treating stress in a patient: 3 drops of clary sage oil; 3 drops of lavender oil; 3 drops of geranium oil; 10mL grapeseed oil. All ingredients should be combined in a dark glass jar and shaken to combine. When applying via massage, the applicant should take a small amount of the blend (about the size of a dime) and rub together in their palms to warm before applying to the patient. Focus the massage on the back and shoulders, which can carry a lot of tension in a person experiencing high levels of stress. If you have more time, a full body massage can provide great benefits to a patient suffering from stress. Apply the same technique to the legs, arms, back, neck, shoulders, feet, hands and head. A comprehensive massage such as this (which can take around 45 minutes to an hour) can ensure the complete relaxation of the recipient as they become fully immersed in the experience. Good results can also be achieved using what is known as the *raindrop technique* which will be discussed further in the later chapter on meditation.

[Find it by clicking here](http://amzn.to/1C5NDCf) or type this link into your web browser:
http://amzn.to/1C5NDCf